How To Be Yourself

Overcome Social Anxiety, Stop Being Afraid of Social Interaction and Develop the Courage to Be Disliked

Antony Felix

Your Free Gift

As a way of thanking you for the purchase, I'd like to offer you a complimentary gift:

- **5 Pillar Life Transformation Checklist:** This short book is about life transformation, presented in bit size pieces for easy implementation. I believe that without such a checklist, you are likely to have a hard time implementing anything in this book and any other thing you set out to do religiously and sticking to it for the long haul. It doesn't matter whether your goals relate to weight loss, relationships, personal finance, investing, personal development, improving communication in your family, your overall health, finances, improving your sex life, resolving issues in your relationship, fighting PMS successfully, investing, running a successful business, traveling etc. With a checklist like this one, you can bet that anything you do will seem a lot easier to implement until the end. Therefore, even if you don't continue reading this book, at least read the one thing that will help you in every other aspect of your life. Grab your copy now by clicking/tapping here or simply enter http://bit.ly/2fantonfreebie into your browser. Your life will never be the same again (if you implement what's in this book), I promise.

PS: I'd like your feedback. If you are happy with this book, please leave a review on Amazon.

Introduction

'We are what we repeatedly do. Excellence, therefore, is not an act but a habit.'-Aristotle

You may think of someone who is successful in life and has attained excellence as being lucky, but the truth is, his/ her excellence is a habit he/ she has built over time. Excellence too, like success, is a relative term and means different things for different people, but generally, when defining it, we do take into account the element of confidence, courage, self-acceptance and self-respect. Those who have these character traits are likely to be successful in whatever they do and achieve their goals, whatever they are.

All of us pursue excellence and success in one or the other way, and in this pursuit, we often come across numerous hurdles, both from the external environment and from within. The external obstacles are certainly tough, but it is primarily the internal problems that keep you from being yourself and your finest version which is exactly what you need to be happy and successful in life. If you do not feel good about yourself from within and experience stress, anxiety and insecurity constantly, you won't be able to move forward smoothly in life.

Being anxious when you have a real challenge to overcome, or when you see hell breaking loose for real is normal and our body's innate response to cope with the situation.

However, if anxiety is your go-to emotion for all times especially the minute you find yourself in a social situation, you are likely to struggle a lot in life. No matter how much you try or want, you cannot stay confined in a single room and cannot excel in life without interacting with people. It is one thing to be an introvert and take pleasure from being with yourself and a few people you feel connected to; or not to want a huge social circle, but even then, you need to have the confidence to socialize and communicate with people.

Social anxiety is a menace that can keep you from being yourself, interacting with people, communicating effectively with them, doing what you want and taking a stand for things you believe in. This is one gigantic internal obstacle that you MUST overcome if you wish to be happy, peaceful, successful in life and strive for excellence. That said, often, people find it quite a challenge to accomplish and struggle with overcoming their inner demons that constantly demean them and feed on their strength, courage and confidence. Fortunately, with this guide by your side, you can actualize this very goal successfully too.

Created with the aim to help you empower yourself, this handy guide provides actionable information and potent techniques on how to understand, accept and acknowledge your condition, dig deeper into it and then consistently and tactfully work on managing your issues to 'dissolve' your anxiety with time, and ultimately become self-assured and strong. In the end, you will accept yourself, embrace your uniqueness and focus on polishing it instead of shunning it.

When you feel happy being you, you only grow more confident and peaceful with time which also gives you the courage to face people and socialize with them.

After reading this book, you will feel motivated to improve on yourself so you can take full control of your life for real and steer it in the right direction. You will feel good in your skin, but also be stimulated to become stronger, let go of your inner demons and overcome the habit of trying to please people so you face them with strength.

So what are we waiting for? Let us get started with this guide so you too can start living with a smile on your face.

Table of Contents

Social Anxiety- What It Is And How To Identify It

Are you scared of being around people?

Does being in a social situation, particularly one where most people are strangers, make you feel highly nervous and agitated?

Are you a very self-conscious around people and that makes it difficult for you to be comfortable in even ordinary social situations?

Do you feel all eyes are on you when you go outside?

Do you often find yourself trying too hard to please others in order for them to like you and perhaps lower your anxiety levels?

Do you struggle with being who you are because your nervousness and apprehensiveness takes over you every time you are in a social situation?

Do you often cancel on meet-ups and get-togethers just so you do not have to meet people?

Do you often experience great difficulty in understanding your emotions and accepting them?

Do you struggle with saying and doing what you want because you lack self-confidence?

If you answered to even a few of these questions and have started feeling uncomfortable again and have been feeling this way for over a couple of months consistently, it is likely you suffer from social anxiety disorder and are quite frustrated with yourself and your life.

And the truth is, you are not alone; social anxiety is the most common of all forms of anxiety with most people ranking the fear of being around people or being judged negatively higher than the fear of death (in simpler terms, some people would rather be the ones on a casket than the ones to speak before people to give the eulogy!).

Let's take the discussion further to gain a better understanding of what this disorder is and how you can identify it.

Understanding Social Anxiety Disorder

Social anxiety disorder, also referred to as social phobia, is a mental health disorder, which entails persistent and intense fear of being constantly watched, scrutinized and judged by other people.

If you experience social anxiety, this can be a strong fear that tends to influence your everyday life, your attitude, your feelings and beliefs, your relationships and your academic and professional life as well. It can make it really tough for you to feel comfortable and peaceful in life, as well as carry out even the simplest of tasks especially those that require even the littlest of involvement with people.

Feeling nervous in some situations, those involving and not involving people is perfectly okay. For instance, you are likely to feel apprehensive when going on a date with someone you have had feelings for a long time, or when pitching your business plan to a big group of potential investors, or when you feel you are slipping into a financial crunch. Experiencing nervousness is quite natural in those instances.

However, if anxiety seems to persist (for days, weeks or even months without going away, especially during any social situations you find yourself in, what you may be experiencing is not normal; it leans more on social anxiety disorder. This is when you feel anxious being around people and strongly (even if you know it is irrational) believe that everyone you encounter is judging and belittling you. You become highly self-consciousness, and this makes it incredibly difficult for you to behave normally and peacefully.

Here are some of the commonly experienced signs and symptoms of social anxiety.

Do You Really Have Social Anxiety Disorder? The Signs & Symptoms

Your level of comfort in different social situations tends to vary depending on the type of people you interact with and the kind of social situation you find yourself in. Some people are naturally more outgoing and extroverted while others are more reserved and shy.

That said, shyness does not symbolize social anxiety and a lack of confidence. In contract to the normal nervousness one experiences when meeting people of different kinds, social anxiety disorder is different as it encompasses avoidance, apprehension and a strange fear that interferes with your routine tasks and functioning. The disorder mostly begins in early to mid-teenage years, but can also commence sometimes in adults or in children below 12 years.

Behavioral and Emotional Symptoms

The signs and symptoms of social anxiety disorder include the following:

- Fear of being judged: If you have social anxiety, you feel that everyone around you has all eyes on you and is constantly judging you. Even if nobody is looking at you, you sense a pair of eyes piercing your heart and judging every ounce of your existence. This feeling alone tends to weigh you down and cripple you emotionally.

- Constantly worrying about humiliating yourself: This fear of being constantly judged is rooted in the worry of doing something that may humiliate you. You worry that you will embarrass yourself and in case you do something embarrassing, others may judge you which weighs you down.

- Intensified fear of socializing with or simply talking to strangers: You find it impossible to talk let alone socialize with others because your mind is constantly fixated on the belief that you will make a fool of yourself and that others are judging you.

- Fear that everyone will notice your lack of confidence: You are also likely to fret over what may happen if others sense your inner fears and make fun of that.

- Avoiding speaking or doing anything you want to comfortably because you fear embarrassing yourself: All the fears stated above cripple you emotionally and this can greatly drain your courage and confidence. When you don't feel self-confident, you do not easily and comfortably voice your thoughts and do what you really wish to do.

- Fear of showing physical symptoms that may give away your anxiety: Lack of confidence makes it difficult for you to accept yourself and your condition which almost makes you feel guilty for feeling that way. This makes you fear the thought of showing any physical symptoms that may make others notice your anxiety. If you blush, tremble, sweat or have a shaky voice while speaking, you are likely to become even more upset and anxious because you know others will notice your apprehension and judge you for it.

- Feeling extremely anxious anticipating a certain event or activity: Your fear is not just associated with how you feel about yourself or how you think others perceive you, but it can also come from thinking about a certain important activity or event, particularly one that involves any sort of interaction with people. For instance, you are likely to find yourself in a pool of anxiety if an important board meeting is coming up in your workplace or right before a seminar in college that you ought to attend.

- Spending a great amount of time analyzing and scrutinizing your performance after being in a social situation: You are also likely to spend a significant amount of time analyzing and primarily scrutinizing yourself after being in any sort of social situation, be it big or small. Whether you just went out to the supermarket to do grocery or went to your friend's football match, you will spend hours thinking about how you behaved, what you did, how you stood or sat, the way you spoke and how others reacted or responded to your behavior even if all you managed to get was a mere glance from someone sitting next to you. Your performance evaluation won't just be about important events because it is likely you won't speak or do something at a large scale. You are likely to keep worrying about the everyday situations and even that will cause you truckloads of anxiety.

- Always expecting the worst outcome associated with a situation or event: When thinking about an event or a situation, your mind jumps to the worst case outcome instantly. You leave out the good or even the neutral outcome and go straight for the worst and most terrible things that you think are likely to happen to you. If you are going to take an exam, you know you will fail in it. If you are going to showcase your startup at a trade fair, you are positive nobody will even show up at your stall. Whatever the situation is, you are 100% certain only the worst outcome will be your fate.

With these emotional concerns, apprehensions and symptoms come some physical signs and symptoms as well.

Physical Manifestations of Social Anxiety Disorder

If you are prone to experiencing social anxiety, you are often likely to exhibit the following symptoms of it.

- Fast heartbeat
- Blushing
- Sweating
- Trembling
- Nausea
- Upset stomach
- Indigestion and heartburn
- Shortness of breath
- Taut and tensed muscles
- Blank state of mind
- Lightheadedness
- Dizziness
- Neck and shoulder pain
- Numbness in a body part mostly your limbs

If you are susceptible to social anxiety, the emotional, behavioral and physicals signs and symptoms are likely to affect you every time you are in a social situation. This makes being in a social situation and any new environment unbearable for you so you start avoiding even the most routine social situations and experiences such as:

- Going to the supermarket to do grocery

- Making small talk with strangers or unfamiliar people outside in a store, mall, when buying something or standing in a queue

- Going to your college or workplace comfortably

- Starting a conversation with someone and maintaining it

- Conveying your message to someone

- Giving an answer to a question asked from you thinking you may give the wrong answer and embarrass yourself

- Attending any social event, even a party

- Dating

- Eating comfortably in front of someone

- Returning an item to a store or asking for an exchange

- Requesting for a favor from someone

- Entering a room full of people where mostly people are seated already

- Using a public restroom

- Speaking loudly in a crowd so others can hear you

- Telling someone he/ she is wrong even if you know you are right and even if the disagreement is petty and won't result in any grave consequence

You need to observe yourself and your behavior for these signs, symptoms and manifestations of anxiety. If you note even 4 to 5 of these behaviors and manifestations consistently over 4 to 6 weeks, and their intensity only seems to increase with time, you have social anxiety disorder.

Yes, it does go away or lessen in intensity when you avoid social situations, but this does not solve the problem. Your anxiety will only intensify and may turn into depression if you do not address it effectively right now. The next chapter shares with you the first strategy you need to employ to become empowered and battle your anxiety issues.

Know What You Must Do And Why You Must Do It

There's just so much going on in my mind, sometimes I can't keep up with what's going on around me." - Amanda Jade Briskar

If you experiencing a racing mind every now and then, the quote above will resonate with you.

There probably have been many instances in life when you felt your mind would instantly explode because there was a barrage of thoughts running wild everywhere and you just did not know what thought to focus on, what to pick and what to let go of. You could not focus on anything else, were not even aware of what went on the outside, did not even realize the actions you were taking because your thoughts would not let you rest or pause for a second.

Anxiety does make your life feel chaotic and wreaks havoc in your head, which then leads to disruption in your life. It is not a very pleasant feeling, especially when it sabotages you emotionally, physically and psychologically.

That said, it is important to take the right route to work on this issue in order to deal with it appropriately without blaming yourself, feeling guilty or nurturing any sort of negativity for yourself.

Here is how you can go about that route sanely, peacefully and nonjudgmentally.

1: Accept Something Isn't Right and It is Anxiety

For a lot of anxiety victims, the mere act of realizing and accepting that they have a disorder to tackle is extremely overwhelming and this often keeps them from acknowledging their problem.

This is also rooted in the stereotypical and judgmental behavior of the society towards mental health issues. Someone with anxiety, depression, any type of OCD or PTSD is referred to as 'crazy', 'lunatic' or 'mental' by those around us. Instead of understanding and accepting a mental health problem as a glitch/sickness of the mind, which is just like a physical ailment such as fever, diarrhea or typhoid, people perceive mental health issues as a declaration of someone's insanity.

Naturally, when the society is unwelcoming towards those battling mental health issues, the victims nurture an unaccepting attitude towards it as well. They too feel they are crazy for having certain thoughts or beliefs, and if they dare share it with someone else, they will only be made fun of. Considering this, it is understandable if you too do not nurture a positive attitude towards your mental problem and shun it every time you feel there is something serious that needs your attention.

However, keep this one thing in mind: you are your only ally and the most supportive friend you can ever have. If you do not take care of yourself, nobody else will. This is how the world works and the sooner you accept this reality, the better. It is okay if nobody around you understands your problem, or labels you as crazy. It is sad, but okay.

What's more important is that you need to stand for yourself and that will happen only if you acknowledge your problem.

Acknowledge Your Social Anxiety Disorder

Now that you are well aware of the signs and symptoms to look out for, observe your behavior very closely for a week or two. Get a supportive and trustworthy loved one on board in this mission too if you feel comfortable with this idea right now. If there is someone who cares about you deeply, he/ she will be ever ready to lend you a hand. If, however, you are not ready to share it with someone else, no problem.

Just do what makes you feel comfortable.

- Write down the anxiety signs and symptoms on a piece of paper and every time you observe any of those symptoms in yourself, circle it.

- You need to note the duration for which a certain symptom persists, its frequency and the timing of its occurrence.

- Also, note down what, in your opinion, must have triggered it. Every bout of anxiety you experience is set off by something. It could be the thought of going to study in a new city; the controlling behavior of your friend; and the fact that you cannot stand to be around people even though you do wish to have a nice, comforting social circle.

- When you experience a certain anxiety symptom, notice how it makes you feel and if possible, write down those feelings (immediately is fine and if you can't record them immediately, later is fine).

- You need to go through that account before going to bed or at any other time if doing so before your sleep time makes you more anxious.

- As you read a sentence or recall a symptom, think of how it made you feel and say 'I accept I felt/ feel this way' very clearly and loudly so you hear it ring in your ear. Try to do it at a time when nobody is around so you feel comfortable confessing it. Repeat this suggestion on every symptom.

- Analyze the current state of your life and if it is not what you had in mind for your life, understand that your anxiety is one of the reasons behind this undesirable manifestation.

- Solidify your acknowledgement of your condition by saying, '*I have social anxiety disorder and it is okay. I accept my condition and myself, and am going to put in consistent efforts to feel better.*' Your acknowledgement can be worded differently too, but remember to keep your statement as positive and accepting as possible. Notice how none of the words in the statement above are judgmental or discomforting because we understand how even a single unaccepting word can set off a torrent of chaotic thoughts inside your head and trigger your anxiety. Keep this in mind and be as gentle as possible with yourself.

You are likely to feel both overwhelmed and liberated when you make this declaration, but it is okay. Just do not react to anything you feel and you will be okay. If tears trickle down your eyes, let them do so. If you feel perspiration dance on your forehead, let it run its course. If you do not react to it, you will feel okay; in fact much better with time.

2: Know Why You Must Work on Assuaging Your Anxiety

After accepting you have a problem to deal with, you need to pump up enough motivation inside you to take the step forward. Any goal that you set in life *must always be accompanied by compelling reasons that stimulate you to act towards it*. The importance of having compelling reasons to pursue your goal cannot be emphasized enough and there is a strong reason why.

On your pursuit of a certain goal, there will come times when you would not want to move even a step further. There will be times when you will only be gasping for air and would want to give up on your pursuit that very instant. There will be times when you will feel the goal has lost its charm for you. Does that mean you should stop moving towards that goal then? No, of course not! If you strongly feel connected to a goal, you should always pursue it no matter what, but you also need to prepare yourself for times when your motivation starts to deplete. This is where the compelling reasons come in handy.

Your 'why' attached to your goal comprises of all the compelling reasons why you must pursue that goal and stick to it no matter what. When the going gets tough and you don't see your goal anywhere in sight, it is these reasons that remind you of what you are trying to chase and why you must keep at it. These very reasons provide you with the strength, motivation and stamina needed to persevere in tough times and do not surrender to fears, setbacks and despair at any cost.

Your commitment to yourself to cure your social anxiety disorder is quite a huge goal, one that you can obviously accomplish with hard work, consistency and perseverance, but one wherein you will at times stumble and find yourself engulfed in frustration. In all such times, the compelling reasons to overcome your social anxiety disorder that you draw out right now will help you out and will put you right back on track.

Here is what you need to do.

Draw a Comparison between What is and What Can Be

To feel obligated to work on your goal, draw a comparison between how your life is right now and how you want it to be. Close your eyes and think of how your life is right and what you do not like about it or wish to change.

- Think of all the times you start sweating with fear the minute you step into a room full of people.

- Think of how you feel all eyes are on you and how uncomfortable that makes you feel.

- Think of how you do not spend any time with your loved ones because you are constantly engulfed in your worries.

- Think of how you are constantly having fights with your partner because you do not feel like going out with them because of your anxiousness, and he/ she is tired of staying locked in the house.

- Think of how you have to settle for what others decide for you only because you are scared of voicing your opinion.

- Think of all those times when your fear of not being liked by others makes you act as their slave and go against your wishes.

- Think of all the times when you lack belief in yourself and aren't able to pursue the things you wish to do.

- Think of the times when you so wanted to talk to someone, but could not because you were unable to muster enough courage to do so.

- Think of how your colleagues at work keep taking advantage of you because you feel too weak to stand up against them for your rights.

- Think of how you stay indoors for days even when you so wish to get some fresh air and meet friends.

- Think of how you keep missing out on trainings, workshops and growth opportunities at your work because you are too scared of interacting with people.

- Think of how your inner demons keep sabotaging you from within and every day you find yourself growing weaker emotionally and psychologically.

- Think of how your dreams, aspirations and ambitions are slowly vanishing into thin air because now you do not even feel like dreaming let alone pursuing those dreams.

- Think of how with each passing day your body aches, neck pains, stomach problems and other physical issues are only increasing.

- Think of how you feel a storm of emotions wreak havoc inside you and leave you crippled in every possible way.

It is okay if you feel overwhelmed when writing down these observations or even thinking about them. If it gets too unbearable for you, stop the session right there and carry on after a few hours or the next day.

When you feel better, think of how you actually want your life to be. Think of how you want all of these issues to be resolved and enjoy the following:

- Feel emotionally stable and relaxed

- Feel self-confident and poised

- Feel peaceful in your skin and not constantly demean yourself

- Feel okay to not feel okay

- Feel physically fitter and healthier

- Find it comfortable to go outside and be in social situations

- Easily start conversations and maintain them

- Compliment people when you wish to

- Disagree with people without fearing they might hate you

- Maintain your stance and stick to your viewpoint without any inner fear

- Believe in yourself, your capabilities, strengths, skills and potential and constantly improve on it

- Go wherever you want, however you want

- Stop worrying about things beyond your control and focus only on improving yourself

- Accept, embrace and love yourself

- Feel comfortable with your loved ones

- Strengthen bond with your loved ones by focusing on their needs

- Improve workplace performance and productivity which helps you enjoy better growth related opportunities in your career

- Attend parties, gatherings and meet-ups whenever you want to

- Focus on your health, wealth, abundance, happiness, relationship, success, career and spirituality related goals with a relaxed, stress-free mind

- Feel anxious only when you are supposed to and not every other minute of the day

- Talk to people easily and comfortably

- Stop feeling that others judge you

Just imagine for a few moments how your life would be if you are able to achieve all these outcomes. The peace, tranquility, serenity and mindfulness that would enter your life then is surely going to be priceless and will only add value, meaning and empowerment into your life.

Naturally, when you feel confident in yourself and feel okay even if people dislike you, you won't get the urge to please them or budge from your stance when you don't wish to. This helps you take your decisions yourself and manifest an empowered life for yourself.

Every day, for about 15 to 30 minutes, you need to imagine achieving all of these outcomes and enjoying them. Add details like sights, expressions, emotions, colors, sounds and textures in the imagination to engage all your five senses in the experience. This engrosses you in the imagination making it more vivid for you. This immerses your subconscious mind in the imagination thus helping it embrace the suggestions easily. The minute your subconscious mind accepts something, it makes you focus on the goal and work in that very direction. That is how you employ the power of your subconscious mind to actualize all your goals and overcome social anxiety disorder for good.

Do this daily and you will feel extremely motivated to curb your anxiety and live a more peaceful, meaningful life for good. With this motivation and commitment, you are now ready to move to the next strategy to further your progress.

Be Mindful Of Your Emotions And How The Environment Affects Them

Social anxiety victims mostly feel that others around them, particularly strangers, are staring at them and judging them. The truth however is that those people are shining that light on themselves- they are just as anxious as you may be. Since it is now established that you have social anxiety disorder, it is highly likely that you too have a habit of shining too much light on your own self. While you feel others are staring at you, it is you yourself who is doing that deed.

That said, you won't realize that because you are not mindful of yourself and your emotions at all. You are so engulfed in your anxious thoughts that you fail to pay even the littlest attention to how you actually feel and what induces those emotions. This lack of awareness also keeps you from comprehending the real reasons behind your anxiety.

The thing is; anxiety has pretty much become a part of your life, but there are factors that set it off. It does not come from nowhere, but has certain triggers, which you may not even be aware of. This unawareness is a huge reason why you have allowed your social anxiety to get out of control and make you feel uncomfortable in your own skin. It is quite likely there are certain situations or instances that set off your anxiousness, but since you aren't aware of them, you may stay in that situation for a long time only to let your condition worsen. If you are mindful of yourself, you will soon be able to get better control of your anxiety and find it easier to accept and love yourself.

What Mindfulness Does for You

A study published in the 'Social Cognitive and Affective Neuroscience' Journal states that mindfulness affects the areas of your brain involved in stress and anxiety. Participants of the study with moderate levels of anxiety experienced around 39% reduction in the overall anxiety levels after going through mindfulness based training.

There are countless other studies that validate this and prove that mindfulness does wonders to your stress, anxiety and even depression related issues. Research from the University of Amsterdam suggests that mindfulness is not only an effective, but also a very accessible and cost-effective method to soothe and treat social anxiety disorder, as it provides anxiety victims with more control over their ability to focus and understand their thoughts and pay attention to the techniques they employ to resolve their problem.

Mindfulness basically refers to living in the moment you experience fully, completely, peacefully and nonjudgmentally. Mostly, we aren't really present even when we are present and that's because we are only physically present, but not emotionally and mentally. You may be doing a task, but your thoughts are likely to be elsewhere and if you do pay attention to what you are doing, you seem to be judging and labeling it especially if you are prone to social anxiety. That's why you may just be talking to your friend, but in your head, it is likely you are thinking about how your friend may be judging you or that you should not have said certain things.

Instead of just focusing on the conversation, you are constantly thinking about what may happen, what did happen and how you made mistakes just now. This keeps debilitating your self-confidence and you only fall deeper into the trap of your anxiety. If only you are mindful of the very moment you are experiencing, you are likely to overcome anxiety due to the following effects:

- You will focus only on the conversation and how it makes you feel. If it makes you feel happy, you continue with it; if, however, it brings about ill feeling, you excuse yourself from it to curb the ill feelings there and then without aggravating them.

- You become aware of your emotions instantly and respond to them appropriately by seizing the moment and doing what you know will help you feel better.

- If you do slip into anxious thoughts, you learn to gently bring back your thoughts to the moment at hand without judging yourself or your thoughts.

- You do not label any emotion you experience in the moment or the situation you encounter as bad, negative or ill. Yes, something may be undesirable for you, but you accept it as it is without thinking negatively of it. This keeps your anxiety from worsening because when you embrace things as they are, nothing really upsets you too much. When your anxiety isn't set off, you are able to maintain your calm even when going through a rough situation.

- You do not rehash the past and thinking of anything that happened and this in turn keeps your anxiety in control. You also do not think of any unfortunate event that may happen and worsen your condition. By doing this, you only focus on the present and each moment that flows one after another- which keeps you grounded and focused on the now only.

All these changes are precisely what keeps you cool, poised and focused, and help you slowly steer clear of the vicious cycle of anxiety. You start to understand that it is 'you' who keeps shining the spotlight on yourself by thinking of old occurrences where maybe you embarrassed yourself or made a mistake and someone pointed you out which is why you worry incessantly about what may happen if you repeat the same mistakes.

You also understand that others may not even be aware of your presence, but since you overthink stuff, you associate different thoughts and feelings to others because you aren't aware of how you feel. You also understand how you ignore the root causes of your social anxiety, which is why it only increases with time. Moreover, you become aware of how you must compel your mind to be mindful of the very moment so you can seize it and enjoy whatever the moment brings forth for you without worrying about anything else because this moment will never return.

These realizations help you become more peaceful, accepting and happier with yourself and your life.

Now that you are aware of what mindfulness can do for you, let us take a look at what you can do to attain it.

Mindfulness Based Breathing Meditation

Meditation is by far the most effective and easiest way to inculcate mindfulness because it brings your awareness to the moment and calms down your thoughts.

When your racing mind slows down, you get some time in between your thoughts and this can greatly help you focus better on what you wish to understand.

Here, it is important to stress that your mind functions in 5 brainwave states. Brainwaves are produced by your brain when the neurons in it communicate with one another and the waves are in the form of synchronized electrical pulses. Whatever your mind does (even at a subconscious level), different kinds of brainwaves are created and vary according to your activity, mood and feelings. Every brainwave is of a certain frequency and produces certain effects on your body and mind. The slower brainwaves make you feel slow, exhausted and tired whereas the fast ones make you feel active and alert.

To better understand how meditation induces mindfulness and helps treat social anxiety, it is important to have awareness of the 5 brainwave states your brain mostly functions in:

- Alpha waves: These are the brainwaves you experience when you start meditation or when you enter a deeper state of mind and have a frequency ranging between 8Hz and 12Hz. They calm down your nervous system, lower your blood pressure and regulate your heartbeat. Moreover, they promote relaxation and decrease the production of stress related hormones, which in turn calms you down. Meditation helps your brain easily function in the alpha state when you wish to so you quickly calm down, become focused and relax when you need to. This helps you think things through, focus on what you want, become more aware of your emotions and slowly move out of the social anxiety loop.

- Beta Waves: Your brain functions in this state when you work on a goal oriented task like reflecting on an issue or planning something. They have a frequency range of 12Hz to 30Hz and improve your concentration, create awareness, enhance logical thinking and also help you become a better conversationalist. However, you are able to experience these benefits only when the beta waves work on their optimal level. An overactive beta state induces anxiety, emotional issues and even depression. A major reason behind your heightened state of social anxiety could be your overly active beta state. This is likely to be the reason why you overthink stuff and keep pondering on only how people judge you and nothing else. To feel better and look after your needs, you need to regulate this state which is where meditation comes in handy.

- Theta Waves: These waves are mostly associated with awakening one's third eye, as they help you tap into your spirituality, intellect and wisdom. They induce a positive state of mind, nurture creativity, improve your problem solving and analytical thinking skills, increase your focus and promote calmness. It is this state your mind works in when doing routine tasks such as driving, folding clothes, doing laundry etc. They have a frequency range between 4Hz and 8Hz. Regular meditation slowly helps your brain operate in this state when required, which in turn helps you to turn off the racing state of mind and experience a more relaxed and calm one.

- Gamma Waves: These waves are linked with laser focus and help you experience more positive emotions as well as reduce depression, fear and anxiety. They have a frequency of over 30Hz. While you need to function in an active gamma state when carrying out important tasks so you focus better on them, an overly active gamma state induces anxiety and depression problems, and can even lead to OCD. Mindfulness based meditation can help stabilize the extremely intense gamma waves so you can take a break from all the excessive thinking and relax for some time.

- Delta Waves: These are high amplitude brainwaves with a frequency range of 0Hz to 4Hz. This is the brainwave state your brain functions in when you enter deep sleep. The delta waves improve the production of melatonin and DHEA, which are anti-aging hormones that help you slow down fast aging. Moreover, they help you nurture empathy and compassion for others which enables you to resolve conflicts between people and also improve your bond with loved ones. Meditation helps your brain function in the delta waves, which improves your level of understanding and compassion not only towards others, but also towards your own self. This helps you slowly accept yourself, be your unique self and stop feeling the need to impress others which improves your anxiousness.

Studies show that meditation increases the volume of gray matter in the frontal area of your brain, which improves your emotional stability and focus. The frontal lobe is associated with analytical thinking, critical analysis and active planning. If you have an overly active frontal lobe, you overthink stuff, which only heightens your social anxiety. Meditation helps switch off your frontal lobe so you stop thinking actively at all times and just detach yourself from everything else and relax.

Meditation also slows down the activity of the part of your brain known as thalamus. The work of the thalamus is to relay sensory and motor signals to your cerebral cortex, which in turn improves your sense of calmness. It also slows down the activity of your parietal love which slows down your thoughts giving you time between them and ultimately focus better. The reticular activity, which keeps your brain focused and highly alert is also slowed down by meditation and this improves your sense of calmness.

This is precisely what meditation does to your brain and this in turn calms it down and switches off your ability to feel anxious even when you are not required to. While there are many ways to meditate, an extremely simple and effective technique for beginners is to practice breathing meditation.

Here is how you can do it.

- Sit or lie down comfortably on a chair, couch or on an exercise mat on the floor in a quiet, peaceful nook in your house or a room where nobody distracts you for some time. Being prone to anxiety, it is likely that clutter distracts you and triggers your anxiety. In that case, it is even more important to relax in a clutter free and organized room, as this ensures you do not feel anxious after every few seconds.

- Close your eyes and think of any happy memory or anything that calms you down. Keep thinking of that object or memory for a few minutes until you feel more emotionally stable and relaxed.

- When you feel better, slowly and gently bring your attention to your breath. To do that, just let go of any one thought you are thinking about and observe how you inhale through your nose. As you inhale, do it in your natural way without deepening your breath, but ensure to do it through your nose.

- When you inhale, observe how the air moves around in your body, makes your tummy flatter and makes your abdomen rise. Notice the little to more noticeable sensations in your body thanks to your breath to stay focused on it. You may not observe anything at first, but if you keep at it, you will start to sense them and become more engaged in the practice.

- After a few seconds, when you are ready to exhale, let go of any other big chunk of thoughts from your head and exhale through your mouth. This time, focus on how the air moves out of your body into the air producing certain sensations in your body during the process.

- You need to keep breathing in this manner and stay focused on your breath throughout the process.

- During this time, you are likely to find yourself wander off in thought. Maybe the thought of the tasks lined up disturbs you, or maybe you keep thinking about how you need to pick your son from school and that is likely to upset you. Whatever thought pops up, distract yourself from it without bringing in any sort of judgment. You can count your breath loudly or in your head to divert your attention from the distracting thoughts. Just keep doing it and you will feel a lot more focused and relaxed within a few minutes. It can, however, take you more sessions than one to get your focus straight, which is perfectly fine. You have just started to train yourself to be mindful which is why you may take some time to get there, but you will reach that point if you stay consistent with the practice.

- For about 2 to 5 minutes, even 10 minutes in the start if you can meditate for that long in the start, you need to keep inhaling and exhaling consciously while closely watching your breath. Set a timer for that duration so you don't keep peeking at your watch or phone to keep track of time every few seconds and disrupt your practice.

- When the timer beeps, very gently and slowly open your eyes. In every mindfulness based practice, what you need to remember is that everything must be done slowly and gently, as this greatly helps you to become more involved in it and work on the task consciously.

You then need to register your feelings and emotions when the practice ends and you are likely to feel quite relaxed, focused and grounded. Hold on to these emotions and return to your other chores with that frame of mind so whatever you do, you do it with a peaceful and conscious state of mind. It is advisable at this point that you build a habit to journal your thoughts and feelings after every session of mindfulness based breathing meditation and draw a comparison between your anxiousness before and after the session. This helps you keep track of your anxiety with time.

After practicing mindfulness based breathing meditation a few times, you will find yourself becoming more mindful of your thoughts in the routine. This awareness slowly gives you better insight into the root cause of your social anxiety and helps you figure out your anxiety triggers. When you are aware of what switches on your anxious mode and what makes it persist for hours and days, you will then be able to bring changes to your routine accordingly to manage the triggers. For instance, you may realize that your social anxiety was first triggered when you were bullied in high school by friends you trusted a lot. Now that you know being bullied turned on your social anxiety, you can then look for such instances and occurrences in your everyday life that keep reminding you of that instant and worsen your condition.

You need to constantly keep track of your feelings and emotions through your practice and the ability to stay mindful. With time, you will sense anxiety bubbling up inside you the minute you feel anxious in a social situation. When you realize you are feeling anxious, you then take account of your thoughts that very moment. It is likely you are overthinking something, probably something that isn't true and when you acknowledge that, you can then easily bring your attention to the moment through your breathing. Make sure to consistently practice mindfulness based breathing meditation regularly to become more aware of your breath and the present moment through it. In addition, work on the following techniques to improve your state of mindfulness as well.

Mindfulness Based Walking

Walking is one thing we do a lot throughout the day. When walking takes up a good part of your day, it is understandable that many of your thoughts brew up in your head during that time.

So you are walking down to the dry cleaner and you keep thinking about how the passerby is staring at you and finds you weird; or you are walking towards the kitchen, but cannot stop thinking about how you have to present something in front of your bosses in a meeting tomorrow.

This just shows that you aren't mindful at all when you walk or do anything else for that matter.

To inculcate complete mindfulness, you must stay aware of your thoughts and emotions, and the actions those thoughts and emotions make you take at all times so you can quickly curb your anxiety by responding appropriately.

This can happen successfully if are mindful of your thoughts while walking.

Here is how you can do that.

- Every time you get up to walk and do a chore, take one step forward consciously. If it helps, say '*I am getting up and taking a step forward.*'

- When you take the next step, say 'I am putting my left foot forward' and just keep doing that until you reach where you had to.

- Be conscious of how your foot feels on the ground, how you put your foot forward in front of the other one, any sensations in your legs and how the complete act of walking makes you feel.

- Even if it is 10 steps that you take towards the bathroom, be conscious of those 10 steps and your thoughts along with that. You may think of this as a small thing, but you will be amazed at how easily it keeps you mindful of your thoughts with every step you take and in general as well.

You need to make this a constant practice so that every time you get up, you do not allow any unnecessary thought to corrupt your mind. In so doing, you let go of every meaningless thought that had occupied your mind earlier, and keep your thoughts focused on the present only. In a matter of days, you will start feeling more in control of your thoughts and this will help you curb your anxiety and become more peaceful.

Mindfulness Based Eating/Cleaning/Working

Just like you trained yourself to walk mindfully, you need to slowly inculcate the habit of doing every single thing very cautiously. Whether you are cooking, cleaning, eating, reading, working on a project, talking to a client, creating a design or doing anything else, you must do it very carefully so you do not give your thoughts any room and chance to go anywhere else.

In so doing, you ensure you don't give mindless thoughts the power to pollute your mind and distract you from the present.

- Always say out loud the name of the task you are doing. If you are going to have a meal, say 'I *am going to eat a bowl of spaghetti and meatballs.'*

- Visualize the task in your head and then take the first step. If you are going to have your lunch, take the first bite very slowly and very gently put it in your mouth. If you are typing on your laptop, pay attention to how your fingertips touch one button after another and the sound that produces.

- Keep focusing on every tiny detail very thoughtfully to become more involved in the task. When eating, pay attention to the aroma of the food, take bites slowly, chew them even more slowly and feel how the chewed bite moves down your throat. When cleaning a table, notice how the rag moves on the table and clears one speck of dust after another.

- Stay observant of everything as you do and try to take more interest in the task as you carry it out.

By following the ideas above, you will start staying more conscious of your thoughts and will soon realize that if you actually do everything cautiously, you will have very few things to worry about because you do not give your thoughts the opportunity and time to worry about anything else but the task at hand.

Mindful Listening and Observation

In addition to doing every task with increased attention, slowly train yourself to become a mindful listener and observer of everything around you. You may not realize this now, but if you reflect on your everyday behavior and feelings, you will realize that about 80 to 90% of the times, in your everyday routine, you listen to things and observe with a general bias in your mind.

It is the biased thoughts that make you think strangers in the mall are noticing you. It is the bias that makes you believe that if you utter a word, you will only embarrass yourself. It is again the biased thoughts that make you only notice the taunt in your friend's tone if he/she points out your mistake, but not the concern he/ she has for you. When we listen to or observe something, we do so mostly with a preconceived notion glued to our mind. This preconceived notion is what makes us nurture certain beliefs, many of which are often untrue which then make us react irrationally towards things, people and situations.

By training yourself to listen and observe things mindfully, you slowly inculcate the ability to perceive things for what they are without attaching any preconceived notion to them. If you are standing in a crowd and notice the man standing next to you frown, you understand that he isn't frowning at you, but possibly on some thought that popped up in his head. If you are chatting with your colleague, you focus only on his words and not the constant chatter in your head that suggests your colleague hates you or is scheming some sort of plan to ruin your reputation.

This helps you keep your thoughts clear of any unnecessary and pointless clutter and only focus on your wellbeing and the moment at hand.

To develop this ability, do the following:

- Pick any song that you have never heard before and listen to it with a clear, relaxed and nonjudgmental state of mind. Ensure to pick a song by an artist you neither like nor dislike so you do not attach any judgments to it. Play it and just go with the flow. Focus on each word, every beat and every tune, as it enters your ears and do not think of anything as good or bad; just listen to it for what it is. Shun any judgments if they enter your realm of thoughts casually by only focusing on the lyrics and tune of the song. Keep doing this for the entire length of the song and in just 2 to 3 sessions, you will realize that you were never really listening to things acceptingly in your everyday life.

- Just like mindful listening, practice mindful observation by choosing any natural object you wish to explore, such as a leaf, a ladybug, the moon or anything else. You need to observe it with a relaxed state of mind and pay attention to it from different angles. If you are observing the moon, look at the visible patterns you see and analyze them without thinking of them as ugly or beautiful. Focus on how the moon beam reaches you and how it makes everything it falls on shine. Just keep observing your chosen object very cautiously and immerse yourself in the experience by concentrating on tiny details and engaging your five senses in it.

Every day, or at least 3 to 5 days of the week, you need to work on the two aforementioned techniques for 5 minutes each to clear your head of any preconceived notions and learn the art of mindfully observing and listening to everything. After practicing these techniques, you will feel far less anxious in any social situation because you will remind yourself of how you must not attach judgments to your feelings and perceive things for what they are.

Staying in the Moment without Judging Your Emotions

We have talked several times about not judging your emotions, perceiving them for what they are and living in the moment acceptingly, but what exactly does that mean and how can you implement it in real life?

What it really means is to observe an emotion with an open and accepting state of mind and perceive it only as an emotion and nothing else. For instance, if you feel angry, you accept your anger as an emotion you experienced in response to something upsetting without labeling it as positive or negative.

The labels given to your emotions determine your reaction towards it. So if you perceive your anger as something negative, you will feel bad about it, which may make you anxious and in turn continue to think negatively. Similarly, if you don't feel confident in a situation, but belittle yourself for it instead of embracing it, you will only feel more nervous and may suffer a panic attack.

Just like you have learned to perform normal and important tasks with increased mindfulness, you need to extend this level of consciousness and understanding towards your emotions. Every time you feel a certain emotion, register it by taking a break from whatever it is you are doing and focusing on the emotion. Think of what exactly you are feeling and then accept it by saying or writing, *'I am feeling anxious/ envy/ sad etc. and I accept my emotion.'* Saying it out loud helps you register it verbally and by writing it down, you solidify your acceptance towards it.

Once you have accepted you feel a certain emotion, try to understand it with empathy. Ask yourself questions such as: Why do I feel this way? What is this emotion trying to tell me? Do I actually feel this way or am I overthinking things? Is this a genuine emotion or something I picked up on from someone? People who are susceptible to social anxiety have a tendency to pick up emotions from elsewhere. It is likely this happens to you as well. Asking these questions helps you explore the emotion nonjudgmentally.

As you experience the emotion, do question it, but do not put any label on it. Your anger, envy, sadness and frustration is just an emotion like your happiness, peace and contentment and it will too pass if you do not hold on to it. Every emotion you experience, especially if it is a strong one intensifies for a few seconds and then fades away provided you don't hold on to it. So if you do not hug your anxiety tightly, it will slowly diminish. When you experience it or any other emotion you do not wish to continue experiencing, just accept, acknowledge and explore it and let it intensify and then subside on its own.

In those times, try not to react by taking an impulsive action in response to that emotion. If you feel anxious, excuse yourself from the situation and just sit with your emotion instead of running away or locking yourself in a room. If you experience a panic attack, try to avoid yelling in response to it and look for a quiet corner where you can sit peacefully and understand your anxiety. Yes, this will be hard to do, but responding to your emotions is precisely what helps you manage them effectively and appropriately, and equips you with the ability to treat them as emotions and not as 'war sirens.'

Once the emotion subsides on its own, recall the entire experience and think of how you behaved. Also, think of suitable ways to tackle the problem if there is any and the right way to respond to your emotion. If you were upset about something which triggered your anxiety, how do you think you should respond to it? Tackling the problem when the dynamic emotion has surpassed is the right way to go about resolving your issues and mitigating your social anxiety.

Now that you are aware of how to inculcate mindfulness through different practices, ensure to do this every day to slowly make mindfulness a constant part of your life. It will soon become a habit and you will start staying in this very state all the time. With this ability, you will also find it easier to achieve progress through the other techniques that will be taught later in the book. Let's move to the next chapter to find more helpful techniques.

Relaxation Techniques

A relaxed body and mind is crucial to feeling good about yourself. If you feel shaky from within, are exhausted and physically and emotionally swamped, your mind is likely to wander off in gazillion places and make you feel even weirder, anxious and disturbed than how you feel right now. Oftentimes, anxiety stems from stress that hasn't been dealt with appropriately or at all. For instance, your increasing workload with each passing day may be stressing you out which may make you feel nervous about your performance and your boss's attitude towards you. If, however, you successfully turn in all the projects on time, you are likely not to feel that anxious.

An effective approach to tackling your social anxiety and reducing routine stress is to relax yourself on a regular basis.

Here are a few techniques, which, if you carry out on an everyday basis, can soothe your anxious and exhausted nerves so you feel comfortable and slowly overcome your fear of interacting with people.

Practice Body Scan Meditation

Body scan meditation is a powerful relaxation and meditative technique can help you unwind, calm your stressed out body and mind, and nurture a more positive relationship with your body. Sometimes, social anxiety is also rooted in a lack of comfortable and accepting relationship with your body.

You may have been body shamed for a major part of your life, which may make you think you aren't good looking. This consequently may make you feel not confident in your skin and also believe that others judge you.

By developing a healthier bond with your body, you feel better about yourself and this can greatly improve your perception of your body and your self-image. Naturally, when you start to accept and like yourself better, you feel comfortable moving in public as well and stop nurturing negative thoughts about yourself.

To enjoy these benefits of body scan, here is what you should do.

- Lie down flat on your back on a yoga/exercise mat or on your bed and spread your arms and legs.

- Take a few moments to feel comfortable in the pose and close your eyes.

- When you feel more comfortable, slowly start observing all your body parts, one at a time.

- Begin with observing your toes or any other part of your body you feel the most stress in and would like to observe. If you are scanning your toes, notice any sensations that you feel in them; see if there is any stress in your toes or any heating sensation. Wiggle your toes and see how that makes you feel. You also need to observe how you feel about your toes or any other body part that you are observing. If you don't like it, why is that and what feelings do you nurture for that part? If you do not like a certain body part, accept it by saying, '*I am comfortable with my tummy/ arms etc. and accept it deeply.*'

- As you observe a body part, take deep breaths and imagine any stress in it slowly diminishing. Do this for a few minutes with every part of body and keep addressing every part like this.

- Within 15 to 20 minutes, you are likely to feel a lot more relaxed and peaceful.

You need to practice at least once daily to get rid of all the anxiousness you have developed over the course of the day. Within a couple of weeks, you will feel more positive about yourself, which will make it a lot easier to experience and endure any social situation.

Japanese Finger Stress Reduction Technique

Stress, if left untreated, can become extremely chronic. The 'Japanese finger stress reduction technique' is a simple and incredibly effective technique that soothes stress and anxiety in only 5 minutes.

Your fingers contain nerves that have nerve endings in your brain and are connected to different parts of your brain. To achieve different outcomes such as peace, confidence, tranquility, happiness etc., you need to activate the sensors in your fingers to stimulate the relevant parts in your brain.

The Japanese stress reduction technique is based on this phenomenon and helps you mitigate anxiety within minutes.

Here's how you can practice it.

- With your right hand's fingers, gently press on to all the 4 fingers and then thumb of your left hand one at a time. Press on a finger gently and firmly and massage it for about 4 to 5 seconds.

- Your thumb helps fend off anxiety, stress and worry. The index finger is associated with warding off your fears; the middle finger enables you to control bitterness and rage; rubbing your ring finger helps you reduce depression and melancholy; and your pinky finger improves your self-esteem and feelings of positivity. When you rub each of these individually, you stimulate these feelings, which make you feel better.

- Lastly, you need to massage your palm for about 1 to 2 minutes to promote overall relaxation and positivity.

- Once you are done massaging your left hand, do the same to your right hand with your left one.

Practice this exercise at least once daily no matter what to build its habit. This helps you cleanse yourself of built-up stress on a regular basis so it does not keep accumulating and turn into something more monstrous.

Engage in Fun, Relaxing Activities

According to experts, engaging in fun, relaxing activities that help you unwind by boosting your serotonin and dopamine levels and reducing those of cortisol in your body improves your mood, confidence and can help you overcome social anxiety. Cortisol is the hormone associated with stress and anxiety so elevated levels of it mean you will feel highly stressed and anxious whereas dopamine and serotonin boost your mood and positivity so high levels of these two hormones help you feel better.

To lessen your anxiousness, you need to engage in activities that boost your serotonin and dopamine levels, but reduce and normalize those of cortisol in your body. Activities such as taking warm baths, painting, drawing, doing music, singing, playing an instrument, taking a stroll in the park, sitting peacefully in the woods, dancing and playing any sport do wonders to your serotonin and dopamine levels, which consequently improves your emotional stability.

If you do not already engage in such activities, it is time you actually start doing that and turn the one-time practices into long-term rituals. Every Monday could be picnic day, Tuesday could be dedicated for painting and Thursdays could be for dancing. Of course, you can keep any ritual you want according to your interests and likes. So pick a few fun activities you enjoy a lot and engage in them on a regular basis. Not only will you feel more emotionally stable with time, but you will also start to enjoy your life more because now you actually take out time for yourself. While you do this, make sure to love and accept yourself because that is surely the golden ticket to anxiety recovery.

Extending Acceptance and Empathy Towards Yourself

Empathy for humanity is something that goes a long way. If you agree with that, you should also accept and understand that this applies to your own self as well. You need to accept, love and embrace yourself just like you would do to a loving friend. Social anxiety does stem from the fear of being in social situations, but that itself is rooted in a lack of self-acceptance and self-love.

It is often when you do not love and accept yourself that you feel not confident, which makes you think that others too would not like you much. This distorted belief is what needs to change and here's how you can do that.

Challenge Your Misleading Thoughts

Your thoughts that mislead you into believing that you are anxious do the trick. Notice how I did not write 'negative thoughts' here because that would again be labeling your thoughts as bad. Instead of calling thoughts that trigger your anxiety as negative, it is better to refer to them as misleading thoughts because actually, what they do is to mislead you into believing that you are feeling nervous which in turn triggers your anxiety.

A good approach to tackle such thoughts is to challenge them and prove them wrong. Since you allow such thoughts to reside in your mind, they settle in and then grow their roots far and wide something which strengthens them. If only you keep them from sowing their seeds, you can dismantle the huge overgrown anxiety plant successfully.

Every time any anxiety triggering thought runs through your mind, hold on to it before it spreads like wild fire and question its authenticity. Ask yourself questions such as: Is this thought actually true? Was there a time I thought and felt differently? Have I ever been in a situation when I did not feel this way? What evidence do I have to support this theory? Is there evidence that suggests otherwise? Make sure to keep the tone of your questions positive so your mind comes up with positive answers to support them.

Your mind is designed to give you answers to questions exactly the way you ask it. So if you ask yourself, 'Why do I feel anxious?', it will give you several reasons to show you why. When you think of all the reasons that trigger your apprehensive behavior, you are likely to experience it again. However, when you ask yourself questions that suggest there is reason to prove your anxiety is just a feeling that will fade away or that there have been times when you felt confident and happier, you will get answers accordingly that will prove your anxious thoughts helping you feel better.

You need to do this every time an anxious thought disturbs you so you can tackle it promptly and on time without allowing it to wreak any havoc inside your mind.

Accept Yourself

With the ability to challenge your anxious, misleading thoughts and that to stay mindful at all times, you can now easily inculcate self-acceptance. Self-acceptance refers is simply the act or habit of accepting yourself fully, deeply and wholeheartedly. You need to accept yourself the way you are if you are to stop criticizing and disparaging yourself, and embrace yourself with your flaws. Naturally, when you feel better about yourself, you can then move on to overcoming your shortcomings, including social anxiety.

Every night, before going to bed, think of your shortcomings and strengths and write them down on a journal. Tell yourself that you accept and love yourself along with all these qualities and inadequacies, and you are happy with yourself which helps you become better. Give yourself a hug and every time you feel like lamenting over your flaws and social anxiety disorder, think of your strengths and use them to feel better about yourself. Soon enough, you will start to nurture positive feelings for yourself.

Control Only What's Within Your Reach

An important aspect of loving and accepting yourself is to understand that you cannot control everything and can only focus on your own self. If you are now aware of how certain people's behaviors turn on your anxiety and you are positive it is not in your head only, it is time to control the way you behave. You cannot expect such people to change because even if they are wrong, they are the ones who decide how they should live. What you can do is distance yourself from all such people. While you need to slowly work on building enough confidence to face anyone you want, there are certain people whose presence alone is toxic for you. It is best to steer clear of such people so you do not absorb their negativity.

Embrace the Idea of Not Being Everyone's Cup of Tea

Those victimized by social anxiety disorder mostly have an urge to be liked by everyone around them. You need to slowly let go of this desire and understand that you are really not everyone's cup of tea. Even the finest of teas fail to impress certain people because they aren't really fond of tea. Similarly, you too need to stop trying hard to please everyone and become courageous enough to be disliked by some people.

Yes, you should not be unkind and mean to people, but if you aren't doing any wrong and still someone dislikes you, chin up and walk gracefully. It is perfectly okay. Just like you may not like banana whereas your friend loves it, everyone else is entitled to his/ her opinion and if someone isn't too fond of you, just detach yourself from that person and focus on your wellbeing.

As you work on these techniques, you'll slowly gain a lot of confidence and strength to be your own unique person, and will find your anxiety levels dropping low. To curb it for good, it is important to finally face your fears. The following chapter teaches you exactly how that can be done.

Face Your Fears and Interact with People

If you are never going to face your fears, you will never overcome them for good. Similarly, if you won't start to be comfortable around people and interact with them, your anxiety is bound to return sooner or later. You have to face them and learn how to socialize for this ordeal to end for good.

Here is how to go about it:

Take Baby Steps

Facing your fears in no way implies that you need to speak in a crowd of 100 people instantly. That won't help at all and will only be detrimental to your newfound peace. The right way to go about is to act like a tortoise. Yes, you got that right: slow and steady to win the race.

Identify exactly the type of social situation that makes you perspire profusely and your mind go insane, and then set small goals regarding experiencing and enduring it. If speaking in front of people scares you, start off by being around people for a few minutes and slowly increase that duration. Next, speak in a group of 2 to 5 people and slowly speak in front of a larger group. Just go slow and steady, but keep taking steps.

Have a Supportive Buddy Around

Ask a supportive friend/ loved one to assist you in all such times so if he/ she sees you losing your confidence, he/ she can quickly calm you down. Also, if there is a familiar face in the crowd, you are likely not to feel as nervous.

Think of the Bigger Picture

Always think of what overcoming your fears will do to you and how improving on social anxiety disorder will change your life for the better. Write down those benefits in bullet points and stick it to your bathroom mirror. Every time, after you shower, go through that list to remind yourself of what you aim to pursue to get going.

Take the Plunge

You have to take the plunge so do not wait for the perfect time to face the music; just do it. After a couple of weeks of working on the strategies discussed in the previous chapters, dive right in and go in a social situation even if it is just going out for grocery. Do it without talking to people and then treat yourself to a little present. Observe your feelings right after; you're likely to feel accomplished. You then need to slowly move on to making small talk to strangers (asking for directions is a good place to start) with time so you can get over your fears.

These tips go a long way if you work on them consistently and track your performance so ensure to journal it.

Conclusion

I hope this book has offered you real time value and has proven helpful in your journey to overcoming social anxiety. What you need to do is to put what you have learned into practice. The truth is; it will seem impossible at first but as you keep taking action (while of course being mindful of your thoughts, your environment, your body sensations and much more), everything will seem clearer and more doable. If you keep taking action, you won't even realize when you stopped being socially awkward or at least you will have figured out how to deal with your anxiety effortlessly.

Do You Like My Book & Approach To Publishing?

If you like my writing and style and would love the ease of learning literally everything you can get your hands on from Fantonpublishers.com, I'd really need you to do me either of the following favors.

1: First, I'd Love It If You Leave a Review of This Book on Amazon.

2: Check Out My Emotional Mastery Books

<u>Emotional Intelligence: The Mindfulness Guide To Mastering Your Emotions, Getting Ahead And Improving Your Life</u>

<u>Stress: The Psychology of Managing Pressure: Practical Strategies to turn Pressure into Positive Energy (5 Key Stress Techniques for Stress, Anxiety, and Depression Relief)</u>

<u>Failure Is Not The END: It Is An Emotional Gym: Complete Workout Plan On How To Build Your Emotional Muscle And Burning Down Anxiety To Become Emotionally Stronger, More Confident and Less Reactive</u>

<u>Subconscious Mind: Tame, Reprogram & Control Your Subconscious Mind To Transform Your Life</u>

Body Language: Master Body Language: A Practical Guide to Understanding Nonverbal Communication and Improving Your Relationships

Shame and Guilt: Overcoming Shame and Guilt: Step By Step Guide On How to Overcome Shame and Guilt for Good

Anger Management: A Simple Guide on How to Deal with Anger

Get updates when I publish any book that will help you master your emotions: http://bit.ly/2fantonpubpersonaldevl

To get a list of all my other books, please check out my author profile or let me send you the list by requesting them below: http://bit.ly/2fantonpubnewbooks

3: Grab Some Freebies On Your Way Out; Giving Is Receiving, Right?

I gave you a complimentary book at the start of the book. If you are still interested, grab it here.

5 Pillar Life Transformation Checklist: http://bit.ly/2fantonfreebie

CPSIA information can be obtained
at www.ICGtesting.com
Printed in the USA
LVHW112148140120
643672LV00001B/248

9 781951 737177